YOUR KNOWLEDGE HAS VALUE

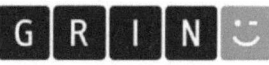

Bibliographic information published by the German National Library:

The German National Library lists this publication in the National Bibliography;
detailed bibliographic data are available on the Internet at http://dnb.dnb.de .

Imprint:

Copyright © 2015 GRIN Verlag, Open Publishing GmbH
Print and binding: Books on Demand GmbH, Norderstedt Germany
ISBN: 978-3-668-20289-4

This book at GRIN:

http://www.grin.com/en/e-book/320377/how-do-breast-cancer-mortality-rates-differ-
between-women-who-are-screened

Amir Hossein Mortazavi Entesab

How do breast cancer mortality rates differ between women who are screened annually and biennially by mammography?

GRIN Publishing

GRIN - Your knowledge has value

Since its foundation in 1998, GRIN has specialized in publishing academic texts by students, college teachers and other academics as e-book and printed book. The website www.grin.com is an ideal platform for presenting term papers, final papers, scientific essays, dissertations and specialist books.

Visit us on the internet:

http://www.grin.com/

http://www.facebook.com/grincom

http://www.twitter.com/grin_com

Table of Contents

Abstract:

Context: Breast cancer is the most common non-skin cancer and second deadliest cancer in women. Mammography, an X-ray of the breast, serves as the primary diagnostic tool for breast cancer detection as it reduces the risk of death through early detection and treatment of the disease. The medical community, however, has not agreed on how frequently such screenings should be performed. [3] Various organizations have produced different guidelines regarding the suggested frequency of routine mammograms. For example, the United States Preventive Services Task Force (USPST) endorses biennial mammography screenings for females ages 50-74, whereas the American Cancer Society (ACS) advocates annual mammography screenings for women beginning at age 40. It is this review's hypothesis that annual mammography is proving to be statistically more beneficial than biennial screening in the reduction of breast cancer mortality rate.

Methods: Full text articles from the U.S. National Institute of Health's Public Medicine's archives (PubMed) were reviewed in order to compare annual versus biennial mammographic screenings and the diagnostic advantages, detriments and mortality rates of each interval.

Results: The majority of articles agree that women between the ages of 40-49 years undergoing biennial screenings are more likely to be diagnosed with late stage disease than women diagnosed during annual screenings. The results for women 50 years and older are less conclusive. While some studies of the over-50 group delineate no difference in the incidence of late-stage disease using either the biennial or annual intervals, the majority of findings suggest the annual interval is more effective than the biennial screening in detecting early stage cancer.

Conclusion: Overall, women partaking in annual mammography screening experience decreased false positive "recall" rates. In addition, earlier diagnoses through annual screenings help detect smaller tumors providing a more hopeful prognosis. While these findings support the importance of annual mammography screenings for women 40 years and older, studies indicate that annual screenings only minimally improve estimated breast cancer survival rates for women aged 50-74 years compared to biennial screening.

Keywords: Breast cancer, screening program, mortality rate, statistics, annual, biennial, frequency, mammography, Risk, American Cancer Society, United States Preventive Services Task Force, late stage breast cancer

Introduction

Breast cancer remains one of the most life-threatening diseases facing American women. Citing the Center for Disease Control and Prevention statistics, approximately 210,000 breast cancer cases and 40,000 breast cancer deaths were reported in 2008.[9] Current statistics show that one in every eight women is diagnosed with breast cancer within her lifetime, and one in every 30 women dies as a result of the disease.[9]

Breast cancer remains the second most common malignancy in females after skin cancer. The disease, which originates either in the ducts or the lobules of the breast, can occur in both human sexes. Two primary categories of breast cancer exist: invasive and non-invasive.[7] The Ductal and Lobular Carcinomas, DCIS and LCIS respectively, are the subtypes of non-invasive breast cancer, while Invasive Ductal Carcinoma (IDC) and Invasive Lobular Carcinoma (ILC) are the major subtypes of invasive breast cancer.[7]

Breast cancer incurrence rates have been associated with three main factors in female patients: advanced age, lower socioeconomic status, and lower education level. Other risk factors associated with the incidence of breast cancer include genetic predispositions, obesity, the use of hormone replacement therapy, and alterations in procreative patterns, for example, the bearing of children at an advanced age or bearing no children. Despite continuing improvements in the diagnosis of breast cancer, over half of the malignancies occur in females whose risk factors are not clinically identifiable.

Breast cancer mortality rates in the United States peaked between the years 1986 to 1991, reaching a high 34% rate. By the year 2007, the number of breast cancer deaths in the United States had dropped to 22%, representing a significant 30% decrease.[1] This reduction in mortality rates is generally associated with the increasing popularity of mammography screening in the 1980s.[1] The medical community references this statistical drop as indicating a strong correlation between early detection via mammograms and improved breast cancer survival rates.

Mammography is generally considered the best diagnostic tool for breast cancer detection. However, the medical community still does not agree on how frequently mammograms should be conducted. Different organizations have released different guidelines regarding the frequency of routine mammograms. For instance, the United States Preventive Services Task Force (USPSTF) endorses two-yearly mammography screening for females between the ages of 50 - 74 years while the American Cancer Society (ACS) advocates for annual mammography screenings beginning at age 40. The lack of consensus regarding optimal frequency for this cancer screen may limit the options available for women seeking earliest detection and treatment. This research attempts to provide significant analysis of the effectiveness of frequency rates, which may lead to lower breast cancer mortality rates.

Rate per 100,000 Females

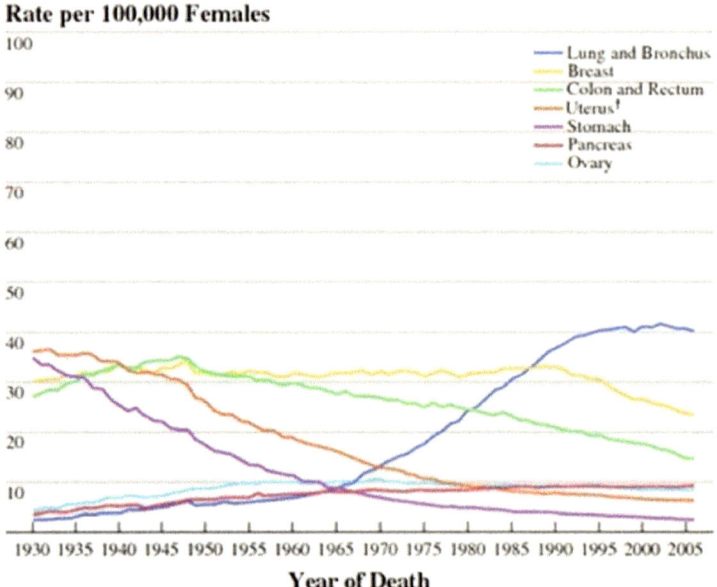

Year of Death

Different malignancy rates among American women, 1930-2006. The graph shows no significant change in mortality from 1930-1990, after which a noticeable decline begins to occur through 2006. (Reprinted from Jemal A, Siegel R, Xu J, Ward E, Cancer statistics, 2010. *CA: A Cancer Journal for Clinicians,* n/a. doi:10.3322/caac.20073)

Methods

Database searched included PubMed, Clinical Queries, Medscape, E-medicine, ACS, USPSTF, Evidence Based On Call, Scientific Electronic Library online, and Google Scholar.

Keywords to search included the following MeSH (medical search) terms: Breast cancer, screening program, mortality rate, statistics, annual, biennial, frequency, mammography, Risk, American Cancer Society, United States Preventive Services Task Force, late stage breast cancer

Publication dates were limited to within the last 15 years; one Canadian published article was utilized.

Study population: Humans, Adult Females

Results

In 2003, the ACS rationalized its guiding principles for early detection of breast cancer on recommendations from acknowledged scientific evidence and research findings. The ACS's most recent screening endorsements include data gathered from test mammography, bodily checkup, the testing of elderly women and women suffering from comorbid disorders, the screening of high-risk females, and precise screening methods .[8] A summary of the current ACS guidelines appears in the table below:

American Cancer Society Guidelines for Early Breast Cancer Detection, 2003 [8]

Women at average risk	Begin mammography at age of 40.[8]
	For women in their 20s and 30s, it is recommended that clinical breast examination be part of a periodic health examination, preferably at least every three years.[8] Asymptomatic women aged 40 and over should continue to receive a clinical breast examination as part of a periodic health examination, preferably annually.[8]
	Beginning in their 20s, women should be told about the benefits and limitations of breast self-examination (BSE).[8] The importance of prompt reporting of any new breast symptoms to a health professional should be emphasized.[8] Women who choose to do BSE should receive instruction and have their technique reviewed on the occasion of a periodic health examination.[8] It is acceptable for women to choose not to do BSE or to do BSE irregularly.[8]

	Women should have an opportunity to become informed about the benefits, limitations, and potential harms associated with regular screening.[8]
Older women	Screening decisions in older women should be individualized by considering the potential benefits and risks of mammography in the context of current health status and estimated life expectancy.[8] As long as a woman is in reasonably good health and would be a candidate for treatment, she should continue to be screened with mammography.[8]
Women at increased risk	Women at increased risk of breast cancer might benefit from additional screening strategies beyond those offered to women of average risk, such as earlier initiation of screening, shorter screening intervals, or the addition of screening modalities other than mammography and physical examination, such as ultrasound or magnetic resonance imaging.[8] However, the evidence currently available is insufficient to justify recommendations for any of these screening approaches.[8]

U.S. Preventive Services Task Force breast cancer screening guidelines

In 2002, the U.S. Preventative Task force, an independent panel of non-Federal experts in prevention and evidence-based medicine, updated the guidelines and recommendations for breast cancer screening. A summary of these guidelines is shown in the table below:

U.S. Preventive Services Task Force guideline for early breast cancer detection, 2002[10]

Women age 40- 49	The USPSTF recommends against routine screening mammography in women aged 40 to 49 years.[10] The decision to start regular, biennial screening mammography before the age of 50 years should be an individual one and take into account patient context, including the patient's values regarding specific benefits and harms.[10]
Women age 50- 74	The USPSTF recommends biennial screening mammography for women between the ages of 50 and 74 years.[10]
Women 75 and older	The USPSTF concludes that the current evidence is insufficient to assess the additional benefits and harms of screening mammography in women 75 years or older.[10]

Other considerations	The USPSTF concludes that the current evidence is insufficient to assess the additional benefits and harms of clinical breast examination beyond screening mammography in women 40 years or older.[10]
	The USPSTF recommends against clinicians teaching women how to perform breast self-examination.[10]
	The USPSTF concludes that the current evidence is insufficient to assess additional benefits and harms of either digital mammography or magnetic resonance imaging instead of film mammography as screening modalities for breast cancer.[10]

A retrospective review cohort study was conducted by Hunt et al. (1999), analyzing over 24,200 women aged 40-79 years in six counties in the San Francisco area between April 1985 and August 1997.[5] The study's purpose was to determine whether annual or biennial mammography best served the public preventative health efforts.[5] The California University San Francisco Medical enter provided a mobile mammography van to screen previously asymptomatic patients.[5]

The collected outcome measures were compared retrospectively for women who underwent annual versus biennial screening mammography.[5] Annual screenings were defined as mammography screenings performed between 10-14 months, and biennial screening included mammography screenings performed between 22-26 months.[5] Screening examinations involved a medio-lateral oblique and cranio-caudual mammographic view of each breast.[5] These examinations were interpreted by board-certified staff radiologists and the interpretations were reported as normal or abnormal.[5] Clinical outcomes for all women with screening examinations interpreted as abnormal were determined by contacting each women's personal physician and by searching the institution's radiology and pathology database.[5] This procedure enabled the researchers to determine the rates of recall, biopsy, and cancer detection for annual screening and biennial screening cohorts as well as the tumor size, lymph node status, and stage of the cancer.[5] A chi-square test was used to compare the rates of recall, biopsy, screening-detected cancer, and stage of the cancer.[5] The Mann-Whitney test was used to asses difference in the size of cancers.[5]

The results are as follow: 518 annual screening recall versus 160 biennial screening recall.[5] The annual screening recall rates of 2.6% was 30% less than the biennial recall rate of 3.7% (P < .0001).[5] 150 annual screening biopsies were performed versus 45 biennial screening biopsies.[5] The annual screening biopsy rate was 0.75%, 28% lower than the biennial screening rate of 1.0% (p = .06).[5] Women who had annual mammography screening showed a significantly lower recall rate (p < .0001) and a lower biopsy rate that approached statistical significance (p = .06).[5] Also the annual screening group exhibited 56% fewer interval cancer cases than those in the biennial screening group (p = .22).[5]

Cancer was detected in 71 women during annual screening versus 19 women in biennial screening.[5] The ratio of screening-detected invasive cancer to ductal carcinoma in situ (DCIS) was almost identical for both cohorts: for annual screening, 75% invasive carcinoma and 25% DCIS; for biennial screening, 74% invasive and 26% DCIS.[5] The annual screening cancer detection rate was 0.36%, representing a 19% reduction compared with the biennial rate of 0.44% (p = .49). [5] The median tumor size of combined screening-detected cancer was 11 mm, 27% smaller than the median tumor size of 15 mm within the biennial screening cohort (p = .04).[5] The mean tumor size of the combined cancers in the annual cohort was 13.3 ± 0.95 mm compared with 18.0 ± 2.19 mm (p = .04).[5] There were also 38% fewer cases of cancer with lymph node (LN) metastasis in the annual cohort group (9/62, 14%) compared with the biennial screening group(4/17, 24%). (p = .37).[5] Evaluation of cancers for +2 stage resulted in 41% fewer cases of cancer in the annual group (14/81, 17%) compared with the biennial screening cohort group (7/24, 29%) (p = .20).[5] Parallel increase in the cancer detection rate with advancing patient age were found within both cohorts.[5]

In addition, White, et al. (2004) conducted an observational study to investigate the effects of annual versus biennial mammography on late-stage breast cancer. The information used in the study was collected from the Breast Cancer Stakeout Confederation (BCBS) that included statistics on more than 4,000,000 mammograms and succeeding cancers.[12] The women included in the study were diagnosed with invasive breast cancer or DCIS between January of 1996, and thirty first of December 2001, with an age range of 40-89 years.[12] Annual screenings were defined as mammography screenings performed between 9-18 months, (median 13 months) and biennial screening were considered to be mammography screenings performed between 18-30 months (median 24 months).[12] Information was collected by mammography registries that participate in the National Cancer Institute funded Breast Cancer Surveillance.[12]

Data was collected from 176 mammography facilities in seven sites across the United States. Information was obtained on the women's demographic and breast cancer risk factors as well as the mammography results for each mammogram.[12] Each mammography registry is linked

8

to a regional Surveillance, Epidemiology, and End Results (SEER) program or to a state tumor registry that provides information on cancer occurrences, including screen-detected and interval-detected cancers.[12] Five of the seven registries (the exceptions are those in California and Colorado) also link to pathology laboratory records.[12] Data collected by all seven registries in the Breast Cancer Surveillance Consortium were included in the study: Carolina Mammography Registry, Chapel Hill, North Carolina; Colorado Mammography Project, Denver, Colorado; New Hampshire Mammography Network, Lebanon, New Hampshire; New Mexico Mammography Project, Albuquerque, New Mexico; San Francisco Mammography Registry, San Francisco, California; Vermont Breast Cancer Surveillance System, Burlington, Vermont; and Group Health Cooperative, Seattle, Washington.[12] The survival rates of breast cancer patients were higher in women screened annually than those of women screened only once in two years.[12]

Cancer was detected in higher proportion in annual screenings, totaling 5400 women in annual screening versus 2440 women in biennial screening (74% versus 62%; P<0.001).[12] Annual screening resulted in 20% DCIS and 80% invasive disease compared with biennial screening that resulted in 17% DCIS and 83% invasive disease.[12] Annual screening resulted in 36% of tumors being less than 10 mm, 42% of tumors 11-20 mm and 22% larger than 20 mm, versus biennial screening which resulted in 33%, 43% and 24%.[12] Both groups statistics do not add up to 100% due to missing information.[12] Annual screening resulted in 36% of identified tumors being less than 10 mm, 42% of tumors 11-20 mm and 22% larger than 20 mm, versus biennial screening which resulted in respective sizes of 33%, 43% and 24% .[12] Both groups' statistics do not add up to 100% due to missing information.[12]

Women age 40-49 years with biennial screening were more likely to have late stage disease at diagnosis than those with annual screenings (28% versus 21%; OR= 1.35, 95% CI= 1.01 to 1.81).[12] There was no increase in late-stage diseases in women 50 years and older in either annual or biennial screening intervals.[12] Among women with breast cancer who were 40-49 years old, a greater proportion of those with biennial screening were diagnosed with late-stage disease. No difference was observed in women 50-59, and among women who were 60 and older; those with biennial screening were more likely to be diagnosed with invasive disease.[12]

Another retrospective study was conducted using statistics from women aged 50-74 acquired from the Screening Mammography Platform of British Columbia (SMPBC) which analyzed the results from mammograms conducted within a two-year period earlier than 1997 and subsequent to 1997.[11] Canadian researchers likened the long-standing impact and 10 years survival outcomes of the two different screenings between the years of 1988-2001.[11] The annual screenings were defined as mammography screenings performed between 10-14 months, and biennial screening were considered to be mammography screenings performed between 20-28 months.[11]

Results of the SMPBC analysis reveal that 0.65% conditions of invasive cancer were detected from the 897,216 screenings. A Cox proportionate risks model was established to foresee the survival of patients.[11] Age, tumor size, nodal status and histological grade were surveyed as potential predictive factors.[11]

Table I Distribution of tumour prognostic factors and corresponding adjusted hazard ratio for breast cancer mortality for 5844 invasive breast cancers diagnosed 1988–2001 in women undergoing screening mammograms through SMPBC (prognostic sample)

Prognostic factor	N (%)	Hazard ratio	(95% CI)
Tumour size (mm)			
1–9	1163 (20)	1.0	—
10–14	1478 (25)	1.31	(1.20, 1.43)
15–19	1210 (21)	1.72	(1.45, 2.04)
20–29	1095 (19)	2.25	(1.74, 2.92)
30–49	480 (8)	2.95	(2.09, 4.16)
50+	224 (4)	3.87	(2.51, 5.95)
Unknown	194 (3)	3.36	(2.43, 4.66)
Lymph node status			
Negative	3608 (62)	1.0	—
Positive	1374 (23)	3.82	(2.91, 5.01)
Unknown	862 (15)	3.36	(2.43, 4.66)
Histologic grade			
Well differentiated	1583 (27)	1.0	—
Moderately differentiated	2074 (36)	1.04	(0.71, 1.54)
Poorly differentiated	1295 (22)	3.42	(2.42, 4.83)
Unkown	892 (15)	3.36	(2.43, 4.66)

CI = confidence interval.

Source: Wai, et al. (2005)

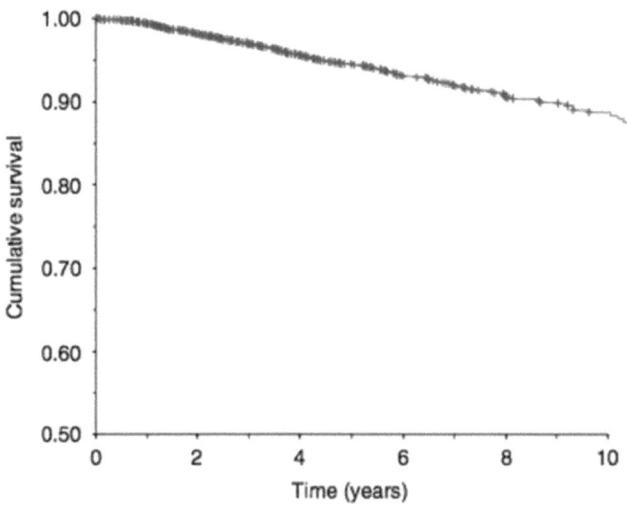

Figure 1 Breast cancer-specific survival rate for 5844 women ever attending SMPBC and subsequently diagnosed with unilateral invasive breast cancer, 1988–2002.

Source: Wai, et al. (2005)

The SMPBC results did not find any significant differences in mortality rate across the women's age span. However, significant differences were detected across other prognostic and mortality factors. This is represented in Table-1 of the article by Wai, et al. (2005). Table-2 of the article shows the dispersal of other prognostic factors representing the 2,441 participants. The predictive silhouette of screen-identified cancer was superior compared to intermission cancers, whereas the silhouette of screen-identified cancers were analogous for women found at yearly or the two-yearly screen.[11]

Findings of the Wai, et al. (2005) research, comparing annual and biennial interval of test mammography in females aged 50-74 years, again showed that an annual interval was superior to the biennial interval as a screening methodology.[11] The five-year survival rate for women screened once per year for mammography was 95.2 %; the rate for women screened once per two years was 94.6% .[11] Similarly, the ten-year survival rate for annually screened women was 94%; for biennial, 89.2%.[11] The five-year difference between the once-yearly screened women and two-yearly screened women was 0.6%. The ten-year difference between the two groups measured 1.2% in terms of survival. Assuming a 100% compliance, this finding corresponds to a 0.89% risk in favor of the yearly screening interval compared to the biennial interval.[11]

Figure 2 of the research article in the Wai, et al. (2005) SMPBC research displays the Kaplan-Meier survival curves for female participants ages 50 -79. The participants had undergone mammography both before and after 1997.[11] No substantial differences appeared in terms of survival rates for women diagnosed before and after the yearly screening interval was adopted.[11]

Table 2 Distribution of prognostic factors among interval and screen-detected cancers in the screening sample

	Interval cancer (%)		Screen-detected cancer (%)	
Factor	≤12 months	12–24 months[a]	10–14 months[b]	20–28 months[c]
Total number of cases (n)	656	655	438	692
Tumour size (mm)				
1–9	11	13	25	28
10–14	19	19	33	28
15–19	20	20	20	22
20–29	26	27	12	14
30–49	11	13	6	5
50+	8	7	2	1
Unknown	5	3	2	2
Lymph node status				
Negative	54	53	67	71
Positive	32	32	15	22
Unknown	14	14	18	7
Histologic grade				
Well	21	21	24	34
Mod	32	32	47	32
Poor	31	31	22	14
Unknown	17	16	7	20
Unknown (size, node, or grade)				
None	25	26	22	26
Any	75	74	78	74

[a]Including interval cancers diagnosed 20–28 months after a screen prior to January 1, 1997. [b]Prior to January 1, 1997. [c]After December 31, 1997.

Source: Wai, et al. (2005)

12

Table 6 Predicted 5- and 10-year survival rates by frequency of screening[a]

Screening frequency	Predicted 5-year survival rate (%)	Predicted 10-year survival rate (%)
'Annual'	95.2	90.4
'Biennial'	94.6	89.2

[a]Predicted breast cancer-specific survival rates based on expected prognostic profile and distribution of interval and screen-detected cancers.

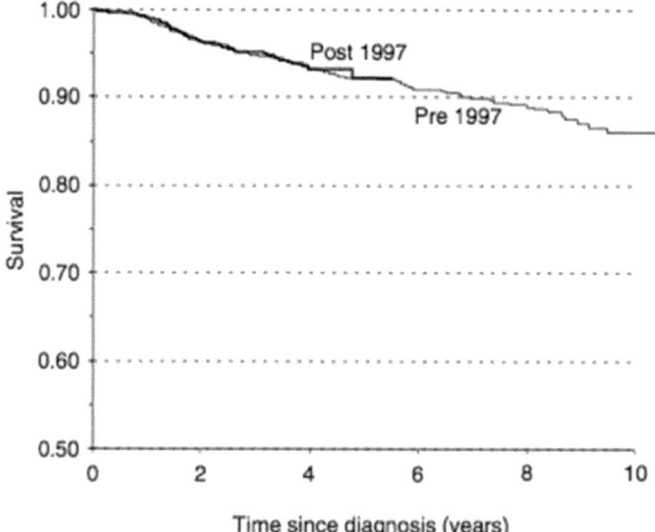

Figure 2 Observed survival curves for women aged 50–79 at screening and diagnosed with breast cancer prior to 1997 (annual screening period) or after 1997 (biennial screening period). Cases prior to 1997 were either interval cases ≤12 months or screen-detected at 10–14 months; those diagnosed after 1997 were either interval cases ≤24 months or screen-detected at 20–28 months.

Source: Wai, et al. (2005)

Discussion

A paucity of data is available for mortality among women screened annually versus less frequently and a controversy exists in regards to the different schedules. The randomized,

13

well-ordered trials which established the correlation of screening mammography to the decrease in mortality rate do not directly address the optimum screening interval.[5] Overall, evidence exists of an increase in advancement of the disease among women with biennial screening versus yearly screening, especially among women in their 40s.[12] Possible contributing factors may include a lack of significant statistics and trials for younger women, a lower incidence of the disease in younger women, and a smaller number of trial participants. However, most studies conclude that annual mammography is the ideal test interval for females between 40-49 years because of the rapid return of the interval cancer rate and an upsurge in the percentage of women with advanced phase breast cancer who had biennial screening schedules.[5, 12, 2]

Based on the study done by Hendrick, et al., using the Cancer Intervention and Surveillance Modeling Network Models of Benefit, annual mammography screening of women 40-84 years shows the highest health benefit with a 39.6% mortality reduction. [4] In women 50-74 years old, annual screening regimens save 71% more lives than the USPSTF-recommended regimen of biennial screening which showed only a 23.2 mortality reduction.[4] For U.S. women currently 30–39 years old, starting annual screening mammography regimens from the age of 40 would save 99,829 more lives than the USPSTF biennial recommendation, if all women comply. Even with the current 65% compliance rate, annual mammography would save 64,889 lives per year.[4]

According to the analysis done by Karla Kerlikowske, MD, a professor at the University of California San Francisco and a medical doctor in the Internal Medicine Department at the San Francisco Medical Center, the highest number of breast cancer patients are women aged 50, mostly white, with dense breast tissue.[6] For women between the ages of 50 and 74, the comparison between those screened for mammography after intervals of three years and two years showed no statistical implication when compared.[6] Women screened biennially between the ages 40 - 49, especially those with dense breasts, showed significantly increased incidence rates of breast cancer compared to those screened annually.[6]

The incidence rate apparently generates some risks as well. Women between the ages of 40 - 49 who undertake the USPST-suggested annual mammography tests for ten years have a greater possibility of receiving false-positive breast cancer "recall."[6] Similarly, in females between the ages of 50 - 74 years, specifically those tested annually for mammography, the false-positive breast cancer incidence rate was higher compared to the same age women screened biennially for mammography.[6]

In the study done by Wai, et al. (2005), women screened annually for mammography had higher survival rates for breast cancer when compared to females tested biennially. The researchers also concluded that no statistical variance existed in terms of survival rates in women diagnosed with invasive breast cancer compared to non-invasive breast cancer. According to Hunt et al. (1999), the cancer with the poorest prognosis is the interval cancer since it occurs between screenings, and women 50 years and older have a slower return of interval cancers, which may suggest that cancer progression is slower in postmenopausal women. So women with increased risk of interval cancer should be on an annual screening schedule rather than biennial screening, to decrease the advancement of the disease and lower the mortality rate in this population. It can be observed that annual mammography screenings result in identification and treatment of cancer with smaller tumor sizes and less lymph node metastasis. Due to early detection, annual mammograms result in decreased findings of stage +2 cancers. Early detection is the most important factor in reducing the mortality rate and the key to a better prognosis.

Conclusion:

The decisions about the strategy might vary from individual to individual based on the risk factors previously mentioned but based on the information gathered for this paper, women partaking in annual screening mammography intervals experience decreased recall rates and an improved chance of identifying and treating smaller tumors with more hopeful prognoses. This analysis supports adopting annual screenings intervals for women 40 years and older. The study indicates, however, that women ages 50-74 do not experience improved estimated breast cancer survival rates by relying on annual rather than biennial screening procedures.

Reference

1.   Cady, B., Michaelson, J. S., & Chung, M. A. (2011). The "tipping point" for breast cancer mortality decline has resulted from size reductions due to mammographic screening. *Annals of surgical oncology*, *18*(4), 903-906.

2.   Feig, S. A. (1997). Increased benefit from shorter screening mammography intervals for women ages 4049 years. *Cancer*, *80*(11), 2035-2039.

3.   Fletcher, S. W., & Elmore, J. G. (2003). Mammographic screening for breast cancer. *New England Journal of Medicine*, *348*(17), 1672-1680.

4.   Hendrick, R. E., & Helvie, M. A. (2011). United States preventive services task force screening mammography recommendations: science ignored. *American Journal of Roentgenology*, *196*(2), W112-W116.

5.   Hunt, K. A., Rosen, E. L., & Sickles, E. A. (1999). Outcome analysis for women undergoing annual versus biennial screening mammography: a review of 24,211 examinations. *AJR. American journal of roentgenology*, *173*(2), 285-289.

6.   Kerlikowske, K., Zhu, W., Hubbard, R. A., Geller, B., Dittus, K., Braithwaite, D., ... & Breast Cancer Surveillance Consortium. (2013). Outcomes of screening mammography by frequency, breast density, and postmenopausal hormone therapy. *JAMA internal medicine*, *173*(9), 807-816.

7.   Mayo Clinic Staff. (May, 2013 22). *Diseases and conditions breast cancer*. Retrieved from http://www.mayoclinic.org/diseases-conditions/breast-cancer/basics/definition/CON-20029275

8.   Smith, R. A., Saslow, D., Sawyer, K. A., Burke, W., Costanza, M. E., Evans, W. P. I. I. I., ... & Sener, S. (2003). American Cancer Society guidelines for breast cancer screening: update 2003. *CA: a cancer journal for clinicians,*53(3), 141-169.

9.   U.S. Cancer Statistics Working Group. (2013). *Breast cancer statistics.* Retrieved from: http://www.cdc.gov/cancer/breast/statistics/

10. US Preventive Services Task Force. (2009). Screening for breast cancer: US Preventive Services Task Force recommendation statement. *Annals of Internal Medicine, 151*(10), 716.

11. Wai, E. S., D'yachkova, Y., Olivotto, I. A., Tyldesley, S., Phillips, N., Warren, L. J., & Coldman, A. J. (2005). Comparison of 1-and 2-year screening intervals for women undergoing screening mammography. *British journal of cancer,92*(5), 961-966.

12. White, E., Miglioretti, D. L., Yankaskas, B. C., Geller, B. M., Rosenberg, R. D., Kerlikowske, K., ... & Taplin, S. H. (2004). Biennial versus annual mammography and the risk of late-stage breast cancer. *Journal of the National Cancer Institute, 96*(24), 1832-1839.

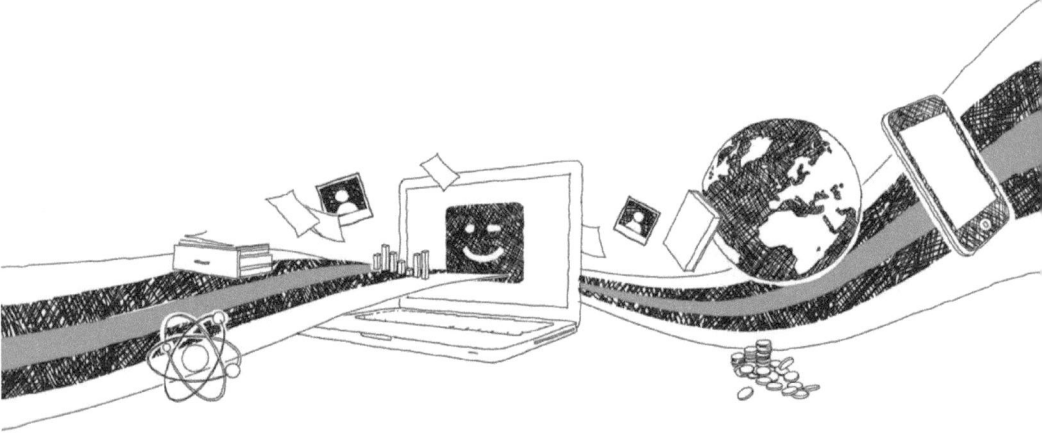
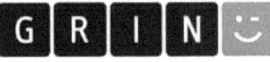